Identifying ADHD:

A Guide to Cultivating Calm, Reducing Stress, and Helping Children Thrive!

© **Copyright 2017 by** _____ **- All rights reserved.**

The following eBook is reproduced below with the goal of providing information that is as accurate and reliable as possible. Regardless, purchasing this eBook can be seen as consent to the fact that both the publisher and the author of this book are in no way experts on the topics discussed within and that any recommendations or suggestions that are made herein are for entertainment purposes only. Professionals should be consulted as needed prior to undertaking any of the action endorsed herein.

This declaration is deemed fair and valid by both the American Bar Association and the Committee of Publishers Association and is legally binding throughout the United States.

Furthermore, the transmission, duplication or reproduction of any of the following work including specific information will be considered an illegal act irrespective of if it is done electronically or in print. This extends to creating a secondary or tertiary copy of the work or a recorded copy and is only allowed with express written consent from the Publisher. All additional right reserved.

The information in the following pages is broadly considered to be a truthful and accurate account of facts, and as such any inattention, use or misuse of the information in question by the reader will render any resulting actions solely under their purview. There are no scenarios in which the publisher or the original author of this work can be in any fashion deemed liable for any hardship or damages that may befall them after undertaking information described herein.

Additionally, the information in the following pages is intended only for informational purposes and should thus be thought of as universal. As befitting its nature, it is presented without assurance regarding its prolonged validity or interim quality. Trademarks that are mentioned are done without written consent and can in no way be considered an endorsement from the trademark holder.

Table of Contents

Introduction 1

Chapter 1: Why is My Child Different? 6

Chapter 2: Is It Really ADHD? 10

Chapter 3: Honing in on My Child's Abilities 27

Chapter 4: How I Influence My Child's Behavior 39

Chapter 5: Where Does My Child Shine? 46

Chapter 6: Developing a Strategy for Your Child 54

Chapter 7: Giving Them a Workable Skillset 68

Chapter 8: Protecting Their Self-Esteem While Helping Them Grow 83

Chapter 9: Bringing the Whole Plan Together 92

Chapter 10: Giving Them Wings to Fly on Their Own 95

Conclusion 98

Description 100

Introduction

Congratulations on downloading *Identifying ADHD: A Guide to Cultivating Calm, Reducing Stress, and Helping Children Thrive!* and thank you for doing so.

The role of the parent is probably one of the most precarious careers in the world. The responsibility of molding the minds of young ones, shaping them into responsible adults, and motivating them to be all they can be can be a daunting one. Even under the best of circumstances, parents are fraught with worry about the right thing to do.

These things weigh heavy on a parent's mind and rightly so. It is perfectly natural to want your child to succeed and take their place in the world. No matter where you come from, what culture fosters you, or even what genetic background forms you, the parents play the most important part of your child's life as their primary guidance counselors.

So, it stands to reason that when a child begins to struggle or loses interest in life in general, is distracted or can't control his emotions it would be a legitimate and necessary cause of concern. The fact that you are reading this book is proof that you are like most other parents in search of answers to the hard questions.

Watching a child who has to fight every day just to perform the most basic of functions that his peers can do easily is hard. It often forces parents to seek for answers in areas outside of their field of expertise and in light of a lack of understanding of the issues affecting their child. Sadly, they often tend to look for these answers in all the wrong places. They listen to the well-intentioned advice of their friends and family, they trust the words of the counselors and teachers at school, and they search blogs, forums, and all manner of websites on the Internet.

While it is with good intentions that these myriads of people try to steer them to their way of thinking, the solutions they offer are often not what your child needs. You've probably already heard many of them and may have even tried some of their suggestions to no avail.

It's just a matter of getting tough with your child

Medication is the answer

The problem is with the school

You're coddling them

Give them rewards

Don't give them rewards

They're just testing you

Chances are, you've tried all of these suggestions, listened to every comment and even tried negotiating and pleading with your child and received little to no positive results in return. Adding to your turmoil, there will inevitably come conflicts at home, and you're dealing with what seems to be an ever growing struggle over household chores, homework, and power struggles with siblings.

Now, you're wondering what is wrong with your child. Perhaps you have heard of ADHD from a teacher or relative who has observed something in your child. Whatever the case, the best solution to the situation is to find out what it is and whether this is what's driving your child's erratic behavior. It is said that "Ignorance is bliss," but that is only true when there is no risk of loss. A parent knows that her best defense is knowledge. The more informed you are about your child, the better equipped you'll be to deal with the issue.

In this regard, you, the parent, are the only one that can shed light on the topic. You may consult with your family physician, talk with school counselors and teachers, even glean valuable information on the Internet but always keep these individuals in their proper place. You know your child, you are the one who knows their weaknesses, strengths, desires, tendencies and the intimate nature of their personalities. None of these advisors – no matter how much knowledge they have – can tell you your child has ADHD without your personal input.

Through the pages of this book, we will help you cut through all of the confusion and give you a clear cut vision of what ADHD really is. We'll point out the tell-tale signs that can help you to analyze your child's own behavior and guide your focus in a direction that will best benefit your child.

In part one, we'll break down and explain why children with ADHD are different and what it means for them. How you can determine your child's own weaknesses and strengths and how your actions actually do have an impact on your children and what they do.

In part two, we'll give you the tools you need to work with your child giving him direction and a plan of action that can and in most cases will lead to success. Like George Peppard used to say, "I love it when a plan comes together," when you have a plan to tackle ADHD head on, then you'll love the affect it will have on your child and by extension your entire family. The reality is simple. The sooner you can pinpoint ADHD in your child and develop a workable course of action the sooner your child can began to share some of those same experiences all children have.

Childhood is a precious time in all of our lives, but if your child is truly struggling with ADHD, then he is likely missing out on many of those golden opportunities. Opportunities that make and shape the person he is meant to be, the building blocks of adulthood. There is no time like the present to give him the tools to master these challenges and ensure that your child benefits from those golden moments that will last him the rest of his life.

There are plenty of books on this subject on the market, thanks again for choosing this one! Every effort was made to ensure it is full of as much useful information as possible, please enjoy!

Chapter 1: Why is My Child Different?

We have all been told that it is unhealthy to compare your child to other children his or her age. However, this can be very hard to resist when you see droves of their peers that seem to be moving through life at a much faster rate. An eight-year-old child that can't remember to bring his books home from school or a ten-year old that can't seem to get through his or her homework without being distracted and pulled in another direction can be a scary thing for any parent to witness.

The ADHD child is often quite intelligent. They have no problem grasping the finer lessons of life and education. This is at times what perplexes a parent with a child that strays from the norm in this way. The child may have no difficulty understanding how to work their math problems, can probably write a student essay in record time, and could likely recite entire passages from a reading assignment.

The first thing one must recognize is that ADHD is not necessarily a learning disability. Many children with this condition have the ability to understand and grasp the intricacies of the world around them. However, when it comes to putting this knowledge into action, there seems to be some type of disconnect. What the child is lacking is not the ability to learn but the ability to perform effectively in their environment.

The name itself often presents some confusion for many in the child's life. Attention Deficit Hyperactivity Disorder gives the impression that the child is merely having difficulty paying attention. However, this is an oversimplified view of what's really happening. Over the last 40 years, much research has been done to prove that ADHD is not something with such an easy fix. It is more than just a child's inability to focus; it also involves the child's genetic make-up, environment, and social interactions. To claim it is just a matter of not paying attention neglects all of the other aspects of the disorder. It fails to identify the many challenges that a child may experience as he tries to fit into a fast moving world that is putting ever-increasing demands on him. This is often the reason that many with ADHD also experience bouts of frustration and anger that can be overwhelming for those around them to deal with.

Identifying the disorder is not always easy. Parents often spoke of taking their children to the doctor and having their concerns dismissed. Even medical professionals may not quickly identify the signs of ADHD. Many are often too quick to see parent's concerns as being overprotective of their child or not realistic about their expectations. Whatever the reason, it is up to the parent to insist on pushing the matter until something is done. Far too often, children are diagnosed with the disorder at a later age than could be. This delay can deprive them of years of treatment that could have put them on the right track much sooner.

Unlike physical disabilities or challenges, the child with ADHD looks perfectly normal, so people often expect him to be able to perform perfectly normal tasks. He walks, talks, and engages with his environment exactly as he should. However, as the years roll by it becomes apparent that something is not quite right. He is either out of control or is completely out of sync with the rest of the world. He has an inability to manage himself, her times, or take on additional responsibilities.

An extension of this behavior becomes evident as a state of depression. No doubt you've already seen evidence of this. A child home from school, head bowed low and their face looking totally dejected. He doesn't wish to discuss what happened during the day and may want to retreat to his room and hibernate. He knows that he is not living up to expectations and as much as he would like to, he is unable to do so it on his own, and he doesn't know why.

Your child is not lacking in intelligence and will soon see for himself that he doesn't fit in with the other children. He knows he can't keep up with the world's expectations of him. This revelation may come from your outward disappointment in him, and his behavior or from comments heard from his teacher's, relatives, siblings or anyone else that he may interact with.

The reality is however that if your child has ADHD, he is different. His brain is in a constant state of turmoil, and it is affecting him in a myriad of ways. Many people will tell you that the hyperactivity is because of eating too much sugar, it's just normal for being a kid, or he just doesn't have any boundaries. While many of these suggestions may be true, they are not the root problem for children with ADHD.

In the next chapter, we will learn how to identify the signs of ADHD and what you should know to get your doctor or other professional to understand and address your concerns. Once you begin to fully grasp the identifying marks, you'll begin to see a picture unfold that will reveal whether or not your child meets the criteria for it. If after reading this next chapter you see these markers in your child, the next step is to get a professional diagnosis to get an official diagnosis. Then you can work with him to create a plan of action that will prove to be a relief for both you and your child.

Chapter 2: Is It Really ADHD?

Now that we have the basics of ADHD let's look a little more closely at what it actually is. Because many are diagnosed during their early school years, the disorder is often viewed as a distinctive learning disability. However, it is much more than that. A better and more accurate description of ADHD should be a developmental disorder that can impact an individual's ability to control the attention, impulses, and level of activity. Still, even that is not a full and accurate description of the disorder.

Fifty years ago, many professionals were opposed to even calling it a disorder but after many years of research, careful clinical studies, and observations, we have also learned that if ignored, the condition can eventually extend to interfere with the individual's will and desire to function in a normal world. They may lose all sense of time and fail to recognize conditions of urgency when they arise.

In the past, people would either blame the parents, telling them that they need to buckle down and not let the child have so much control or they may declare it a rather rambunctious phase that the child will eventually outgrow. Some may even go so far as to declare the child inherently uncontrollable and willful.

The good news is that none of those allegations are true. ADHD is not the result of bad parenting, eating the wrong foods, or a temporary phase that the child will go through. After years of research and study, there is a clinical condition that causes ADHD in many children.

It is important that we point out that in this book, we are focusing on ADHD in children, but it is not a disorder exclusive to young children. Many adults also struggle with the problem as it affects relationships, employment, and finances as it touches on all areas of their lives. However, for the sake of this book, we're only addressing ADHD in children. This is primarily because a child with ADHD that has been given the tools to navigate the challenges of the disorder can grow into well-balanced and productive adults. The earlier the problem is diagnosed, the better they will be able to manage their transition into adulthood.

Still, with all that in mind, we don't want to make the mistake of saying that all children that get distracted from their daily responsibilities are victims of ADHD. The reality is that depending on the age, a short attention span could be normal for the child. So how can you determine if this could be your child's problem?

You could consult with your child's doctor, but that is not always a guarantee that they will take you seriously. All too often, medical professionals are in a mad rush to move patients through their offices and may not readily recognize your concerns. This has frequently been the case when the child has a milder form of the disorder. Parents are often encouraged to just try to "wait it out," "keep them occupied," or "just be more patient with them." While well-intentioned, these words are rarely comforting. If you're three-year-old is struggling to sit in a chair for ten seconds, the idea of waiting it out for the next ten to twelve years can seem quite daunting. It can also destine the child to a life of failure, which will inevitably have a serious impact on his or her self-esteem in the long run. Ultimately, the best thing for your child is to determine if it is ADHD or not as early as possible. One of the best ways to do that is to learn what normal childhood behavior is. This way you'll be able to determine if your child's behavior is falling somewhere outside of the norm.

Dispelling the Myths

Before we get into the many intricacies of ADHD, we need to address many of the common misconceptions about the disorder. We have learned more about this condition over the last few decades than we've learned over the last hundred years. However, unless you're really in the middle of coping with it you're probably not aware of the new understandings that have been revealed through all those years of study and quite likely, those in your circle are still of the misguided beliefs of generations long past. Debunking these myths can help you to fully understand exactly why so many have a negative view of ADHD and how those old ideas have changed.

1. There is no evidence to support that ADHD is a real condition

This argument stems from the idea that if there is no visible or clear sign of damage to the brain that the disorder does not really exist. However, there are quite a few brain disorders that also fit within that description. Down syndrome, autism, and bipolar disease are also conditions that do not show any signs of damage to the brain however the diseases are still very real.

In these cases, the problem does not stem from any disease in the brain but in how the brain actually develops over the years or in how the neuropathic pathways perform. Other cases are a direct result of a genetic anomaly. In the case of ADHD, many cases are the result of small and often imperceptible brain injuries or genetic defects, however, not always. There are many causes that can present themselves from a wide variety of factors that do not show up on a brain scan. These can include:

A. A mother's consumption of alcohol during pregnancy
B. Premature birth

C. Infections during pregnancy

D. Or even trauma

All of these can have a significant impact on the brain's functions during those early developmental stages of the brain.

2.   There is no test to identify ADHD

No, there is no medical test that can diagnose any type of "mental" disorders. This is true in all forms of mental disabilities. However, people do not question evidence that supports a diagnosis of schizophrenia or Tourettes, or any of the numerous anxiety disorders that exist today. These are all very real and very obvious mental conditions that can benefit greatly from early diagnosis and proper treatment.

3.   ADHD is not real because it is only found in the United States

According to statistics, many countries are now recognizing ADHD in their population. Cases are now being reported in many countries including Japan, China, France, and New Zealand. This is not, however, an exhaustive list. Many other countries may report the disorder under a different name, or they may not as of yet have learned of the different ways that it may be identified. Whatever the case, ADHD is a legitimate disorder affecting people in all areas of the globe.

4.   ADHD is overdiagnosed

According to the National Health Institute, the Center for Disease Control and Prevention, and the NIMH, ADHD is actually underdiagnosed making it a contributory factor in many problems in society. They estimate that approximately 60% of children with ADHD have yet to be diagnosed and less than half of those diagnosed are receiving proper treatment. That means there is still a large population of children that are struggling with this problem without the aid of treatment, help or understanding.

The general belief that it is being overdiagnosed is probably due to the improved ability of professionals to recognize the problem and identify it for what it really is rather than following the previous idea that it is simply a behavioral issue or the result of bad parenting.

There is no doubt that there are many more misconceptions about ADHD and what it really is but before we can completely address these issues one must recognize that in the field of science and medication research is still ongoing. The field of neuroscience has made major strides in the last few decades, and we've come to understand more about the brain and how it works than ever before in our history. With that thought in mind, it is imperative that one not hold onto the old myths and ideas that once were believed true and learn about the new knowledge and understanding that countless research projects have revealed over the years.

How to Identify ADHD

While every case of ADHD is different, researchers have determined that there are several characteristics that remain constant in all cases. When you're trying to determine if your child has ADHD you should first look for these indicators.

1. Signs of the disorder appear early in the child's development
2. Their behavior sets them apart from their peers
3. It is pervasive. The condition is not limited to one area of the child's life but affects many areas.
4. It inhibits their ability to perform normal tasks that other children their age can do easily.
5. It is persistent. It does not ease up or get better over time.

6. It is caused by abnormalities in the brain or from developmental issues
7. It is the result of biological factors such as genetics, injuries, or exposure to toxins
8. Evidence of biological or sociological effects may not always be seen

As you learn more and more about ADHD, you'll find that while recognizing it as a legitimate condition does not make it new. It is quite likely that if you look back through your own family tree, you'll find stories and cases of ADHD many years before it was recognized. Listen to family stories about the rebellious uncle, the defunct parent, or the "black sheep" of the family. They will probably tell a tale of finger pointing at the family or some other cause simply because they didn't fully understand what was happening in their mind.

If after analyzing your child's behavior you have come to believe that you are in fact dealing with ADHD you need to look a little closer at the situation. Below are several characteristics you should be noticing in your child's behavior that will help you to decide if you're on the right track.

Limited Attention Span

Notice that the main thought here is not just a matter of paying attention but the ability to maintain their attention span for an extended period of time. This involves much more than focusing on what you have to say, it may include forgetfulness, inability to follow through on instructions, inability to perform tasks to their completion, losing things, constantly distracted, and needing to be continuously redirected, or not able to work without direct supervision.

All of these functions require a sustained attention span. A child may genuinely hear instructions given, she may even start out listening, but the slightest noise or movement in another part of the room can pull her away. She may sit in a classroom and hear the teacher's words, but suddenly her mind begins to drift to something else in her life. This can be even more challenging if there is no genuine interest in what is being discussed, demonstrated, or presented.

This may not be evident at the younger ages, but as the child grows up, more and more will be expected, and if her attention span cannot keep up, she will quickly fall behind and lose out. It is believed that ADHD children's attention spans may lag as much as 30% behind that of children their own age. Translating that into terms a layman could understand, a 10-year-old child could have the attention span equivalent to that of a 7-year-old. It is easy to see how this lack of sustainability could actually be debilitating for children as they are growing to maturity.

Interestingly enough, children with ADHD do not have a problem with filtering information their brain receives. It is not a matter of not understanding what is being said. They seem to function in pretty much the same manner as other children without ADHD, but the challenge for them is that they cannot do so for very long. It is also not a matter of a receiving too much information for the brain to process. ADHD children are perfectly capable of handling any information that other children handle, in the same quantities as well but they do tend to lose interest much more quickly than their peers. After their attention span has been maxed out, their brains will begin to wander in search of something new and more interesting to do.

Reactions

Another factor that is evident in children with ADHD is their distractibility. Interestingly, these children are not necessarily programmed to follow every distraction they sense; they generally respond to the same distractions as any normal child would have, however, it is their reaction to those distractions that is the problem.

For example, a child may be completely focused on his or her classroom activities, and then a car backfires on the road. All the children will respond to the loud noise in the same manner, however, with the ADHD child, once distracted they are less likely to remember the task they were working on and return to the original task. Instead, they may refocus their attention for the moment on something that they may consider to be more interesting.

They also tend to tire and get bored of a task much more quickly than one that does not have ADHD. While we don't fully understand why this occurs, there are several theories that seem to fit. Some researchers have concluded that there is a large section of the brain open to arousal so keeping them motivated can be a challenge while others are of the opinion that the rewards they are working for seem to lose value in their eyes as they progress. Whatever the case, many agree that the ease of falling into boredom appears to be the child's need to seek more stimulation.

These children often need more immediate rewards in order to stay on task. When given a choice they often opt for a more kinesthetic approach to their environment. So, rather than being able to sit and listen to a teacher explain things in class, they tend to want to touch and manipulate objects instead. When the opportunity arises for them to become more physically involved in an activity, they will easily more than they would from an auditory or visual exercise.

Deferred Gratification

It is normal for children to be able to learn how to delay gratification as they grow older. They begin to recognize that if they wait a little longer for their reward, they will usually get something better. However, with the ADHD child, the gratification seems to be paramount in their minds. They may choose to do a little work so they can get some reward rather than a lot of work to receive something better at a later time.

This is an important fact to remember as we develop strategies to help children with ADHD function in this fast-paced world. Having small milestones that are rewarded is more likely to keep them on task rather than removing any distractions to keep them focused, but we will discuss this strategy in a later chapter.

Lack of Impulse Control

One of the most obvious signs of ADHD is the inability to control their impulses. This can be evident in a number of ways. They may be impatient when they need to wait in line for something, they may not be willing to raise their hand in class or wait their turn in a game. From the outside, they may appear to be overly demanding and self-centered forgetting the needs of all other people around them. In reality, it demonstrates their inability to control their initial reaction to stimulus without regard to others.

In older children, they may seem to monopolize conversations, talk over people, or say things that are insensitive because they just haven't been able to slow down enough to think about what their words actually mean.

Takes Shortcuts

ADHD children often look for ways to put in the least amount of effort for the most reward they could get. This strategy of taking shortcuts may work for them in some situations but can present major problems in others.

They are Risk Takers

Because of their lack of impulse control, they often leap into situations where they have not fully considered the consequences. They simply plow full speed ahead and often end up in trouble. Statistics show that children with ADHD are four times as likely to have serious accidents as those who do not. Many of those accidents are the result of impulsive behavior, making decisions without thinking through the consequences.

Hyperactivity

There are cases of ADD where children are easily bored and quickly lose interest in their tasks. However, the vast majority of Attention Deficit Disorders include an element of hyperactivity. It presents itself as too much behavior. When they are distracted, they may find they can't sit still in their seats, they are constantly running, yelling, squirming, touching, and any other physical movement they need to receive the stimulus they seek. In older children and teens, you might see them constantly patting their feet, drumming their fingers, or making the same repetitive motions over and over again.

This hyperactivity also extends to hyperactivity as well. Their reaction to their environment is often not controlled. In situations of anger, they may have louder and more violent outbursts where other children will be more measured. They may say or do things without thinking about the consequences or how it will impact those around them.

Difficulty Following Instructions

The problem of follow through instructions is common in children with ADHD. They may listen to and even write down instructions with the best of intentions when it comes to following them but somewhere along the way, they lose their interest and get distracted. It is important to understand that it is not the child's unwillingness to do what is asked but their inability to keep that task foremost in mind.

They may start out doing one thing and quickly lose interest and move onto something else in the process. In time, they may return to that task and complete it, but it never occurs in a straight line. People with ADHD often have a myriad of incomplete tasks that they hop from one to another. Often it is by sheer luck that one actually gets completed and rare that it will be completed on time.

Work Ethics are Not Consistent

This is not just referring to the constant stop and start of the tasks they do, but it also entails the fluctuating quality of the work. One day they may find that they can do almost any task quickly and easily and at other times they may rush through a task and pay little attention to how well it was developed; the result could be a very low quality even though they have the skills and knowledge to perform better.

This is most likely a by-product of all of the previous symptoms we've already discussed. Their inability to control their impulses, easily distracted, and the urge for more physical stimulus may pull their mind away from the task at hand. They may at one time be fully engaged in the assignment, and at another time something more interesting may be waiting for them so they finish their work quickly just so they can move on to something else.

A New Understanding of ADHD

Likely much of the above information is not new. Even those without a lot of experience dealing with ADHD may have observed these symptoms in a child. However, recent research projects and studies have begun to uncover the reason behind this inability to focus, follow instructions, remember, plan, and act on decisions.

It is not just that a child with ADHD can and does do these things, but it is indicative of a developmental delay in one important element in a child's growth; that of self-regulation.

As children grow older, there are certain abilities they must begin to develop, and one of them is self-regulating. When they are young, they rely on their parents to do everything for them, but soon they learn to dress, brush their teeth, tie their shoes, and feed themselves and so on. In order to do these things, they must learn to regulate their actions on their own. One would not expect a one-year-old to dress themselves, but if the child is five and still cannot put on his own shirt, the parents should be concerned.

Self-regulation, however, is a skill that is not as readily recognized. Most people look to see if the child knows how to do something but ADHD is usually a situation where the child has difficulty doing what he or she knows how to do.

Many are of the opinion that behavior is merely an act of free well. One chooses which course of action to take in any given situation. However, we now understand that there are certain areas of the brain that control our willpower and if that area of the brain has been impacted negatively, the ability to control one's actions can and often are inhibited. Therefore to understand ADHD one must really learn to understand the fundamentals of the will itself. They must come to grasp that the disability is not in the area of skill, knowledge, or perception but the root of it all is an inability to control their will or to maintain self-control.

Chapter 3: Honing in on My Child's Abilities

Before you can understand your child's strengths and weaknesses, you must first understand what normal behavior is for a child. It is true that all children are different, but there is a standard spectrum of age-appropriate behavior that all children should meet. While your child does not need to be in the very top of the scale, they should fall somewhere in the range in order to be considered as progressing normally.

Up until now, ADHD has been identified and responded to base on reactions to the symptoms that each child has. Now that we have a better understanding of what's involved we can better come up with a course of treatment that will benefit both child and adult and help them to better navigate the ups and downs of the problem.

Executive Skills

A term you will need to become familiar with is that of executive skills. Most people will view this term in relation to being able to perform certain executive tasks like running a business or organizational skills. However, this is not the true meaning when it comes to ADHD. While the ability to plan, decide, and perform tasks is definitely a part of it, the focus should be on the word 'executive.' It is the ability to 'execute' those things you planned, decided upon, and want to do.

Every person needs executive skills in their daily lives whether they are conducting a business or not. Even the simplest of tasks require these types of skills. Think about a simple task you might ask your child to do, eating all their food on the plate. To you, it may be a pretty straightforward thing to do but to the child it involves…

1. Choosing the right utensil to use
2. Utilizing that utensil in the right way.
3. Deciding which item of food to put in the mouth first
4. Chewing the food
5. And returning to pick up another item of food.

In normal children, this is usually done without much fanfare, but the ADHD child may see something exciting in the shape of the food and rather than eating it may discover a number of ways to play with it instead. They may lose interest in chewing and swallowing and prefer to spit or throw the food offending others around them. Even if the child is able to function well at the dinner table, there are many other decisions that may affect his behavior. The relationship he has with his siblings, the number of other distractions in the room, and the risk-reward ratio all are part of the process.

A child without ADHD makes a normal progression towards adulthood with little or no problem, but the ADHD child may struggle with this process every step of the way. Every decision becomes a chore from what foods to eat to something as simple and normal as knowing how to comb their own hair and could present a potential minefield. The development of this skill is a gradual process, and it is reasonable to expect that a child will reach a relative semi-adult independence by the time they reach their late adolescent years. However, they will still need to be reminded occasionally as they progress towards adulthood at which point your primary parenting role will reach its end. None of this is possible for the child if he has not yet mastered these executive skills.

Of course, there are several different types of executive skills that a child must develop. These can be viewed from two different perspectives. First, we can look at them from the developmental angle, these are progressive in nature. In other words, the natural order in which children their age learn these skills. You can also view them from a fundamental perspective; in other words in recognizing what they help the child to do.

Likely the easiest way to understand them is from the developmental perspective. Most people recognize and understand the abilities natural to a toddler, a kindergartener, or a primary school aged child. When you know the order in which certain skills are expected in each child, you can more easily identify if your child is falling low on the spectrum. Let's look at each of these skills and how they develop in the average child.

Response Inhibition: The ability to think before acting

Children who have mastered response inhibition are able to make the connection between stimulus from their environment and the associated rewards. In other words, they learn to respond to stimuli according to an expected result. It is a normal response to both humans and animals. However, those with ADHD struggle to maintain control over their actions and often react without thinking without regard to what the consequences are.

Young children are usually able to wait for a short amount of time without getting overly anxious or disruptive while older children are capable of hearing a decision from an authority figure without debating the issue or becoming argumentative.

Working Memory

This is the ability to recall information and connect it to present tasks. It involves bringing past experiences to mind and applying them to current situations. As a child gets older, they should be able to complete more and more complex tasks. A young child may be only able to complete a one or two step task using their working memory, but an older child should be capable of recalling instructions given to them by a number of different people.

Emotional Control

The ability to control emotions while working on certain tasks or waiting for expectations to be fulfilled is difficult for any child. Non-ADHD children usually master this skill and can handle disappointment at a very early age. Teenagers often have to handle all sorts of emotions as they navigate between test taking, heavy homework assignments, and a variety of stress-related incidents in their daily lives and can still manage to get their tasks done.

Sustained Attention Span

Normally progressive children have the capacity to not only pay attention but are also able to extend their attention span for progressively longer periods of time as they age without getting bored or distracted. Younger children should be able to do this for at least five minutes while teenagers should be able to hold their attention for at least one to two hours.

Task Initiation

Children have the ability to get started on a project within a reasonable amount of time without procrastinating. Younger children should be able to start as soon as instructions are given and teenagers should be able to choose a time to start without waiting until the very last minute.

Prioritizing/Creating a Plan of Action

The ability to create a step-by-step plan of action from start to finish on an assignment or a task. This skill also involves decision making in the process. The child must be able to choose which steps are more important and be able to prioritize them in proper order. Younger children should be able to find ways to resolve issues with their peers while teenagers should be able to develop bigger plans for choosing a university or applying for a job without minimal help.

Organization

The ability to create a system to keep their things in order early on. Young children, with a little coaching, should be able to figure out how to organize their room, school supplies, and playthings.

Teenagers should be able to organize their things on their own without any coaching from parents or other adults.

Time Management

Time Management is the ability to determine the best way to make use of their time. It involves understanding how much time they have to accomplish a certain task and find ways to make the best use of it. To accomplish this, they must view time as important and something that should be respected. Younger children should be able to follow schedules and time limits set by adults, but older children and teenagers should be able to create their own schedules to manage the tasks they have to do.

Goal-Directed Persistence

The ability to establish a specific goal and to stay on task until its completion without getting distracted or drawn into more appealing projects. Young children should be able to see small rewards as a powerful enough goal to persist in a project while teenagers should be able to work on a job for a day, a week or more to earn enough money to buy an object of interest.

Flexibility

The ability to adjust their schedules, expectations, and behaviors in the face of changes, obstacles, or other challenges in order to get their job done. Younger children should be able to adjust to changes and obstacles with little disappointment while teenagers should be expected to reasonably adjust their tasks when they are not able to get their first option without fuss.

Metacognition

Every child must be able to stand back and take an objective view of their situation and determine how best to handle it. This is a self-evaluating skill where they take the role of an outsider, mentally step outside of themselves and observe how they are problem-solving and make adjustments accordingly. Young children should be expected to adjust their behavior after receiving constructive input from an adult while teenagers should be able to analyze his or her own conduct in a situation and make the proper adjustments on their own.

Being able to understand these executive skills is paramount to understanding your child's developmental progress. These skills outline the very basic progress that every child should make and while it may not happen at the same time for each child, if your children's peers are steadily picking up these skills and your child is languishing behind the pack it is cause for concern.

Studies have shown that some of these skills happen as early as the first year of a child's life. For example, response inhibition, working memory, and emotional control seem to occur somewhere between the child's first six to twelve months of life. The planning stage develops soon after. You may not readily observe these skills as they develop but you see them when your child begins to communicate to you his needs and wants. He may not be able to speak yet but has learned to communicate, he develops strategies on how he will get you to understand he needs to be fed, he wants his blankie or if he needs changing.

In the second year, children develop other skills like flexibility, time management, and task initiation. They may appear as very simple forms at first but will become progressively more refined as the child ages. Once you recognize that your child is not keeping up with the other children his age you have a decision to make. ADHD comes in two different forms. Depending on which skills they are weak in the child is not able to either *think* correctly or your child is not able to *behave* correctly.

As you analyze your child using these skills as a measure, you can determine exactly what she needs to get back on track. For example, if his weakness is in an area where he is struggling to recall instructions then you can direct your efforts to create strategies that will help him to retrieve those memories when he needs them. If the weakness is managing emotions, then you will find strategies that will give him tools for those areas.

While both types of skills are necessary for development, thinking skills are used to set goals and create the plans of action needed to achieve them. They help them to be self-seekers, finding their own way to getting what they want or need. However, thinking skills can only take your child so far. They will never be able to achieve their goals if they cannot implement the *behavior* skills. A good plan is only that if the child cannot exercise initiative to get started or maintain sustainability to see it through to the end. The two actually work in tandem, one can only do so much, so your child also needs to be able to master both sets of executive skills in order to succeed.

Now that you know these executive skills you should be able to see them as they grow in your child. It is perfectly normal for a baby to feed from a bottle during their formative years but one would think it quite strange if they were still using a bottle by the time they were in school. It is the exact same things with these executive skills. Their impact on your child may not be as obvious as sucking on a bottle, but they are just as important to your child's developing maturity as he grows older.

These executive skills are the key factors used by medical and psychological professionals to determine if a child actually does have ADHD. While you may consult with your doctor about this concern the chances are that parents have already observed these gaps in executive skills and have a pretty good idea that their child has ADHD even before the consultation.

While many may disagree on the degree of absence of these skills, they all seem to have a general consensus that if these skills are lacking, then it is a case of ADHD. Primary skills they focus on are response inhibition, sustained attention, time management, task management, goal-directed persistence and working memory. These are usually the highest indicators of the disorder. Other skills may also be lacking, but these are the ones that are noticed first. If parents have not recognized them then likely they are pointed out to them by their child's teachers and other adults their child may need to interact with.

It is true that the development of these skills can be slow in many children, even those without ADHD. We have even seen some adults that struggle to keep track of their things are always misplacing their keys, or have a hard time focusing on things that are of no interest to them. These weakness actually to some degree are a part of all of us. However, if you witness a child with a string of these skills lagging behind other children or they do not seem to be growing out of them then it is time to do something about it. Others may tell you that it is not important, to just buckle down and get tough or some other cliché that implies that it's something else, but you owe it to yourself and to your child to make sure that they get all the help they need as early as possible so they can mature in a way that ensures their self-esteem remains intact.

Chapter 4: How I Influence My Child's Behavior

Children are learning machines. In fact, we all are. Their sole role in society is to learn their place in the world and adapt their behaviors to fit in those places. Therefore, to address ADHD without addressing the social dynamics surrounding a child is to do a disservice to them. Our children do not live in a vacuum, and so as we take a closer look at this disorder, it is important that we put it in proper perspective.

Of all the social dynamics that a child must learn to adapt to and fit in, the family is the most important. In most cases, the future success of a child with ADHD hinges on how the family responds to his needs. Because of the close interaction with parents, siblings, and others in the household, how well the child develops those missing executive skills can be impacted in major ways.

For that reason, diagnosing ADHD is not as important as how this fact will affect the family dynamics. A diagnosis does not determine how well treatment will be or how the child will overcome the challenges they face. And as parents are the primary caretakers, they will be the ones that have the most influence on the child's progress through the hurdles he has to face with ADHD. With that in mind, every parent must ask themselves how their reaction to their child's behavior will influence their progress.

This becomes a powerful psychological exercise that will not only reveal the weaknesses in your child but your own weaknesses. There is no secret that managing a child with ADHD is no picnic, without their ability to control emotions, follow through on certain tasks, or to even attain to a certain level of independence, the impact can bring out the worst in many of us, especially that of a busy parent.

So, ask yourself just how do you react when you're at your wit's end; when you have tried cajoling, negotiating, yelling, prompting, and bribing to no avail. It is important at this point that you be entirely truthful with yourself because your reaction may be a contributing factor in your child's ability to adjust to this particular disorder.

This chapter is designed to give you a bird's eye view of your family dynamics and how it may be affecting your child. The questions asked can be hard to accept, but if you are open and honest about the answers, you will reap the rewards in the end. Below is a list of questions you should take into consideration.

1. Are you married or are you a single parent? If married, is your relationship a positive one or do you allow the negative aspects to spill over onto your children? Do you see your spouse or partner as a source of support or is it the opposite?

2. Do you work outside the home? If so, is your job stressful and do you at times bring that stress home with you?
3. Does your work bring you professional satisfaction or does it drain you of your energy, leaving you unfulfilled?
4. How do the siblings interact with the ADHD child? How much of that interaction is monitored and regulated by you and what examples have you set for the rest of the family.

It cannot be overstressed that the family dynamics of a child with ADHD is critical in understanding the child and helping them to navigate the challenges they face. Not only do these interactions tend to be more stressful but evidence has shown that these interactions can have a huge impact on a child's psychological state as well. In fact, statistics show that since the disorder can be genetic, there is about a 25-40% chance that a child with ADHD also has a parent that is also dealing with the problem. This increases the problem exponentially for the entire family. Here is how it usually goes...

1. Parents who are already involved in personal problems see their child's behavior as an intrusion on their stressful lives.

The ADHD child's disruptive tendencies are perceived as consuming their valuable time and demands too much from them.

2. Parents then react negatively to the child's conduct in the form of harsh punishments, emotional outbursts, and irritability.
3. Parents may also withdraw supportive words of encouragement, recognition for good behavior, and the normal warmth and love that every child needs.
4. The child then responds in kind, usually in defiance, stubbornness, or some other negative emotion or attitude.
5. The behavior is then reinforced in the parent's mind identifying the child as rebellious or a disruptive influence in the family.
6. The cycle then repeats

It becomes a circle that never ends. The parents are stressed and withdraw affections that the child needs. Then, the child responds to negative input negatively and the cycle repeats. This may occur over and over again throughout the child's lifetime spreading to all other members of the family as well. In the end, you have a family unit that is dysfunctional, and no one is happy.

This is not to say that the parent's actions are deliberate. In fact, many may not even realize that they are doing it, but it is up to the parents to stop the cycle and get the family on a more nurturing and positive track. This can be even much harder if the parent involved is also ADHD.

Difference Between Mother's and Father's Interactions with ADHD

Some parents comment that there is a difference in how a child with ADHD responds to their parents. Often mothers point out that they tend to have more difficulty with their children than the fathers do. There have been several studies done to determine how accurate this statement may be. One study did show that children tended to give more negative responses to mothers than they did with the fathers.

While the reason for this is unclear, there are a few theories that may explain this particular problem within the family dynamic. One primary theory is that in most families the mother is the primary caretaker and as she is trying to reign in the child's self-control and as a result, negative reactions tend to occur. She is more likely to engage in conflicts with the child than the father who takes a lesser role in the managing of ADHD skills.

Mothers also tend to use more verbal skills in reasoning with their child than fathers do. Since children with ADHD generally struggle with language expression, are less likely to respond to verbal guidance and less likely to absorb the instructions given and therefore will quickly get irritated. Fathers, on the other hand, are not usually the ones to spend a lot of time repeating instructions and may be quicker to punish when results are not met. Therefore, one may draw the conclusion that a parent who talks less and follows through quickly seems to be the one that the ADHD child is most likely to respond to.

Interactions Between ADHD Children and Their Siblings

Next, to the parents, the dynamics of the ADHD child with his siblings also need to be carefully analyzed. It is a known fact that children with ADHD are more likely to argue more, fight more, and even get into or encourage more improper behavior than those without. This will inevitably involve more conflicts in the household.

There is no question that it can be frustrating living your life with an ADHD child. It's no wonder that children without the disorder may feel put upon and treated unfairly. This could naturally lead to resentment from siblings in having to share an additional burden of responsibility in the household when they are expected to pick up the slack with chores that the ADHD child has yet to master. There may also be a measure of envy as they notice that the ADHD child gets more attention and help from the parents than they do.

All of these factors can serve as fuel for an already tense situation and if not handled in the right way could lead to major difficulties for everyone.

What Does it All Mean?

It all comes down to one simple fact, having anyone with ADHD in the home can be stressful, but it is even more stressful when it is a child. Living with ADHD impacts everyone in the household so treatment must also include everyone in the household. Dealing with ADHD is challenging in the best of situations, so it's important for everyone involved to recognize this from the start.

In Part II of this book, we'll give you a few guidelines that can make home life easier to deal with as you start your treatment plans for ADHD. The good news is that there is light at the end of the tunnel. If you can bear up under the inevitable levels of stress, you will have to face it will be that much more rewarding when you see your ADHD child grow up to find their place in the world and grow up to be a responsible adult.

Chapter 5: Where Does My Child Shine?

By now you should have a pretty good understanding of which executive skills your child lacks in as well as how your own weaknesses and perceptions can affect their growth. It is inevitable that there will be times when your own strengths will pull against your child's weaknesses and vice versa. There will be times when the two of you can work together because you are both strong in a certain skill set, but there will also be times when your weaknesses will come up against your child's strong point. Still, the worst case scenario is to have to overcome a skill that both of you are weak in.

As you can probably see by now, there will be many challenges yet to face, but in spite of them all, you never want to lose sight of your ultimate goal. How to help your child to shine in this world. One of the first and probably most important steps to accomplishing this goal is to learn everything you can about your child. When you can identify which executive skills he is weak in then, you will be able to lay out a specific plan of action that the two of you can work at together. Simply by doing this, you will begin to see just how to tap into your child's strong points in order to carve out a path that will give him what he needs.

It is sometimes said, "Whenever the door is locked, try a window." The child with ADHD may have to climb through the window in order to achieve his goal, unlike other children who could simply walk through the door. In other words, they may have to find alternative methods for achieving the same goal because of their lack of executive skills.

This will require you to be observant not just of your child and your family dynamics but also the interactions he has throughout the day. If a task is assigned that does not fit well into one of his stronger executive skills, then you may have to find an alternative approach to accomplish the goal. Each time your child is successful, his self-esteem will grow, and he will be more eager to try again.

Many parents hold to the idea that self-esteem comes from showering their child with compliments and praise and while that is warranted at times there is another, more effective way of building self-esteem in the child. By helping them to succeed on their own. Whenever the child is presented with a task that will challenge their limited ability to execute, showing them how to find an alternative approach to the task could do wonders in how they feel about themselves. When they can accomplish the task to the end, they will be more eager to try again the next time a task is expected of them.

This is not always easy to do. At times, you will recognize immediately that the task is not the right match for your child's skills but at other times it may not be so simple. Learn your child's level of tolerance and be proactive in deciding beforehand whenever possible which activities your child has the best chance to succeed in. Those that you know they can't accomplish try to establish an alternative plan of action to ensure that they are successful.

Managing the School Environment

School is one of those situations where it may not be easy for the parent to suggest alternative assignments or for children to get out of doing certain activities. Helping your child to develop flexibility and emotional control can go a long way in getting them to plow through the task they have in front of them. After all, school is specifically designed to prepare the child for life, and very few things in life will be adjusted to one's liking. In these cases, parents and children together will need to develop a strategy to help them adapt to the situation.

To do this, there are several factors the parents must keep in mind.

1. When an assignment requires your child to tap into their own weaknesses in a particular executive skill, it is important that you pay close attention to their emotional state of mind.

It is very important that the parent tries to understand the reason for the emotional change. When a child has a tantrum, avoid thinking it is just an act of rebellion and try to find out the underlying cause. Children tend to behave very differently at home than they do at school when they are surrounded by their peers. They may be too embarrassed to speak up at school, but if you have an open channel of communication, it may be easier for them to let you know what's bothering them.

It has been said by some parents, "The child that needs love the most tends to ask for it in the most unloving of ways." They may not know how to express themselves clearly so you may have to read between the lines, but once you know the root cause of the emotional behavior the better equipped, you'll be to manage the situation and direct the child accordingly.

2. When they appear to be avoiding an assignment or chore, don't conclude they are being lazy or rebellious. They just may not be able to do it.

Children react to situations in different ways and may not always be able to say they can't do something. Some may lash out in anger, others may withdraw into themselves, and others may simply procrastinate and never get started on the task. These are common tactics that are there to let you know there is a problem.

It is the parent's responsibility to look at the task and try to identify which executive skills are needed and why the child is struggling with it. Then you must create a plan of action that will help the child to address the issue.

3. Look at each task and try to decide which executive skills are needed and decide if your child has developed them.

By understanding the task and the executive skills required, you can compare it to your child's weaknesses and strengths. When an assignment requires a number of skills to complete you can try to find the point at which the child breaks the flow. For example, if the assignment is to write an essay for school, go down the list and see which of your child's weak skills is interrupting the work. Is it at the planning stage or at the emotional stage? Is their weakness in metacognition or is it with flexibility?

4. Determine if the difficulty is in the child or is it from the environment.

Sometimes the problem is not in the assignment but in the environment. TV or music playing in the background could add unnecessary distractions that prevent the child from staying on point;

other children may be self-conscious and not able to focus if they are being watched too closely. Some children may require close observation where others may want independence to work on their own. Only you know your child and their strengths and weaknesses.

5. The Sometimey Child

There are those children that can perform a task in one environment while placing them in another environment renders them incapable of functioning. This may be challenging for a parent, teacher, or child to recognize. The child may have mastered the assignment and knows how to do it well, but the challenge comes when the child has to do it repeatedly.

These situations may be organizational where they must clean up their room or maintain a specific record. As the parent, you may have to make some decisions to ensure that you maintain control over the situation. You may choose to monitor the child regularly to make sure that they channel their energies in the right direction or you might opt to allow the child to slip out of the mode for a while and then go back to it. How you manage, it will depend largely on which emotional skills they are struggling with.

6. Find out What Happens When the Child Succeeds

If they are struggling with a task they have successfully completed before then you need to go back and look at what was different. Did you give them more encouragement? Was the environment conducive to what they need to focus? Was the assignment more difficult, shorter, harder, more interesting? Was it broken down into smaller easier to manage pieces? Did they have breaks? There could be a wide number of factors that can interfere with their progress on a particular task. If they have succeeded before then you know, they can do it, so it has to be something else that is triggering the break.

7. Does the child believe in himself?

Sometimes they have the skills needed to perform the task, but for some reason, they don't believe they can do it. There could be a number of things that can strip a child of self-confidence; they think the task is too big; they had tried the same thing before and failed; they have been criticized or bullied, or someone may have tried to help by taking over the job themselves. Whatever the case may be, helping to build up their self-esteem can boost their spirit in amazing ways.

All of this translates into one simple thought. Being a parent of an ADHD child is hard work but if you want to help your child shine in a way that they can be proud of the rewards on the other side can be amazing.

Chapter 6: Developing a Strategy for Your Child

Up until this point, we've concentrated more on how to identify ADHD in a child and how to identify the problems that are part of the life of the family. By now, you should have a pretty good idea of where your child fits in the whole ADHD picture and you've also come to understand that there are strategies that can be implemented to help your child navigate through life's lessons. You may even be breathing a sigh of relief as you realize that your life doesn't always have to be in such chaos as long as you know what your child can do and how to put it into effect.

There is a lot of truth in the expression, "knowledge is power." It's like any person who is struggling with something that is not readily obvious, once they've received a diagnosis they can relax. A diagnosis, in fact, is a kind of validation, a defense against all those naysayers who want to tell you things like 'it's all in your head,' 'you're a bad parent,' and 'it's not a real problem.' I have seen this happen with hidden physical problems as well. People look perfectly healthy, they don't have a visible limp, they don't show any signs of physical ailments, and so people don't believe they have a real problem. But things change quickly when they have a diagnosis. She has lupus, cancer, heart disease, etc.

It is not that the diagnosis solves the issue, but it validates the patient and those who suffer with them. It gives them something to tell the world so they can start to think of your son or daughter in a different way. With ADHD, this doesn't always happen, but it does help. The family members close to the child now have a framework to work in. Parents can switch from seeing the child as willfully disobedient and stop blaming them for their behavior. Siblings also get to see the child in a whole new light.

While all of that is a relief, it is at this point that the real work begins. You can no longer just go through life 'shooting from the hip' when it comes to your ADHD child. The diagnosis does not change the responsibilities and roles in life that each of you has. A child still has the responsibility of learning life's lessons, and the parents still have the job as primary caretaker, provider, guidance counselor, nurse, chauffeur, and so on. It's time to take this to the next level. It's time to create a plan.

As you come up with a workable plan of action, there are a few basic guidelines that you should keep in mind. By following these, you will be able to help your child get the most out of his or her learning experience. Consider these as the building blocks you will use to develop a strategy for helping your child succeed.

Understand that learning will be different

One of the first things you'll have to grasp is that learning will be different for your ADHD child. While children do pick up core subjects of life through instruction their executive skills they often learned through observation of the people and the environment around them.

No one would question that all children learn differently and at a different pace but with the ADHD child, executive skills are rarely picked up by observation. This child struggles to grasp those concepts that are not obvious and pointed out. That means that you're going to have to make sure that their skills are taught. In this process, you will have to make sure that the child understands what behavior is acceptable, what goals they should try to achieve, and what behavior is not acceptable. Then, you can outline for them a plan of action for each phase of the assignment they need to take and explain each one thoroughly.

These assignments should be done under close supervision at first and then gradually fade out your immediate presence as the child grasps the new principles they are learning.

Stay within the Child's Developmental Level

Many parents have expectations that are far higher than what the child can reasonably achieve. They may expect their five-year-old to be able to do the same things as other children their age but if they have not mastered the executive skills needed to meet those expectations it could place them on a straight path to failure.

Parents must first understand what is normal for children their age and then measure their own child's ability against that. The goal here is to match assignments with the child's ability as a starting point and then help the child build his skills from where he is at, not where you expect him to be.

Start with What is Tangible and Move Towards the Intangible

Whenever we teach life lessons, we start with the tangible. Holding a child's hand as she crosses the street, teaching her how to properly hold an eating utensil, or showing them how to wash dishes will eventually lead to life lessons that teach intangible ideas such as cars can be dangerous, proper etiquette is important, and it is important to be clean.

These are lessons that are essential for every child whether they have ADHD or not, however, in the case of the ADHD child, it is even more important to emphasize the tangible. This will require that you manipulate his tangible environment as a foundation for learning those executive skills he is weak in.

Keep in mind that your presence is also a part of the child's external environment. Becoming a constant reminder of things that need to be done is one way, but there are others. Keeping things in front of them can also serve as a visual reminder of things that need to be done. When it comes to tasks, make sure that the assignments given are short and simple enough that they can complete them within a very short amount of time.

You may also control their environment by limiting the amount of external stimulus to keep them from being drawn into too many distractions. Parties should be small and limit the number of excitable activities they can engage in. If they are very small, hold their hands in crowded places and make sure they understand why you need to.

The general idea is that the child will learn first from the external and over repeated experiences they will eventually internalize the lessons and incorporate them into their daily lives.

Incorporate changes in all areas of the external environment

It is not enough to change one aspect of a child's environment. In order for that child to grasp the lessons given to him, the changes have to include more than their immediate environment. Moving a child into a quieter room with fewer distractions may be a good start, but you need to also consider how you interact with your child and making sure she has appropriate monitoring, interaction with others in the household should also be a part of the environmental changes. Changing the dynamics of the task, the environment, and their interactions simultaneously can make it easier for the child to grasp the fundamentals of whatever lesson you are teaching.

Make Use of the Child's Internal Drive to Help Them Succeed

All children have an internal drive that compels them to learn. A rebellious child, therefore, is not just one that fights his parents but instead is a child that has an internal drive and goal that is different from his parents or other authority figures. This drive is found in all children from babies to teenagers. Learn how to use that drive to motivate your child to learn the lessons you want for him.

This can include a number of rewards for them doing what is expected of them or consequences for going against those expectations. This does not mean giving them a reward for something that should become a part of their everyday life. Rewards can be something as small as praise for a job well done or as grand as a vacation.

To accomplish this, you could give the child a list of options. The primary goal is to get the house clean so options could include washing the dishes, vacuuming the carpet, or dusting the furniture. Notice that there is no outside alternative that does not involve cleaning the house; it does not leave the child with an option outside of the expected behavior. Routines like this on a regular basis will eventually be absorbed into the child's mind as part of a normal routine, and in time he will have less resistance to it. It also helps if the entire family is involved in these types of exercises, so the child does not feel that he is being singled out for this particular lesson.

Once the task is completed satisfactorily, they can have the chosen reward.

Match the Assignment to the Amount of Effort the Child Can Reasonably Expend

There are many types of tasks that children will be expected to do but two types of tasks, in particular, that will require the child to put forth extra effort; those they may not be very good at and those they simply don't like to do. These are the tasks the child is most likely going to be reluctant to do and will put up a measure of resistance when asked.

If it is a task that they struggle to do well, your approach may be to break it down into smaller more easy to handle steps. Break each step down to a size that matches the child's ability to put forth the effort. Do not expect more than that first step from the child. When she masters it make sure you praise her for it. This will give her a sense of accomplishment and satisfaction that will embolden her to be eager to take the next step.

The second type of task you will need to address is the one where the child does not like the job given. This could be something like getting homework done or cleaning up the yard. In many households, this is where the child and the parent butt heads. It becomes a struggle for power and can develop into an ongoing battle that will leave both of you frustrated and disappointed.

Remember, your goal is to get the child to complete the task and override his inner feelings of distaste. Keep in mind, this is a task that the child knows how to do but doesn't like doing it. Try to gauge how difficult the task is to the child and while still requiring them to complete it, modify the task, so it is more palatable. Perhaps getting the child to work for 5 minutes and then taking a break. As they become more willing to tackle the job, you can extend the work time to ten minutes, twenty, thirty or more. Sure, it will take a lot longer to get the job done, but it will get done rather than spending that precious energy in an ongoing battle that may never end.

You might find that at a certain point, the constant stops and starts will be more annoying to the child and they will then finish the task in earnest just so they can get on with something else they would much rather do.

If it is an older child, you can ask him to break down the task into manageable steps so that he feels more empowered. If the steps are done accordingly, and the job gets done both the parents and the child will feel very satisfied and have a sense of accomplishment at the results.

Use Incentives as a Motivator

There is a lot of controversy over whether a child should be given rewards or incentives to do what they should do. I suppose it's that old adage that says a child should do what he is told simply because he is a child. However, that argument is contrary to what a parent's role should be. The parent's primary responsibility is to teach the child how to function in today's world as an adult. Therefore life's lessons should revolve around what they can expect from the world around them.

Rarely do adults do things because it is the right thing to do. They go to work with the expectation of a paycheck, they go to the doctor with an expectation that they will feel better, and they take vacations with the expectation that they will have enjoyment and relaxation. Even God-fearing people pattern their lives by the guidelines that state that they will have an eternal reward at some point in the future. This is the way the world works. So, using incentives to motivate your child to do a certain task fits right in with helping them find their place in the world.

As we pointed out before. This does not mean that an elaborate reward is required for every task. Some children will be motivated enough when they hear a word of praise while others may need a little more incentive to get them to do those harder tasks. By expecting the child to complete the task before the award is given is also a teaching mechanism. It teaches them to delay their gratification, and that working is the only way for them to receive whatever it is they want. No doubt, this is a valuable skill that every child needs to learn regardless of their abilities.

The Support Should Match the Need

This may seem like an obvious one, but it is a little more difficult than you might imagine. Every parent struggles with knowing when to intervene and help their child and when to stand by and let them push ahead on their own. While your heartstrings may pull you to jump in and do something it seems like the child can't do on her own, it is not usually the best course of action.

We've all seen those parents that do their children's homework assignments, hover painfully over their every move and jump in whenever the child begins to falter. These children rarely progress to the point of independence. They grow up expecting everyone to do things for them and rarely put forth any exertion to accomplish goals themselves. As a parent, you want to manipulate just enough, so the child learns what is expected of him.

For example, a child that is learning how to walk gets up and falls down repeatedly before he learns to balance. A parent may stand over him, holding onto his hands and may nudge him to make a step by pushing his legs against the child's in a walking motion. Eventually, the child will understand what walking is and will tentatively take a few steps on his own. In this way, the child learns to walk. The parents help him to stand by holding him up as he learns how to balance himself. Later, the gentle nudging helps him to understand how to take steps first one leg and then the other.

But what happens if every time the child tries to stand and falls, the parent runs in and swoops him up in their arms and comforts him? That parent has interrupted the learning process. Parents should be close in case the child needs assistance but far enough away that he can make a move on his own. Ideally, parents should be there as an observer until the child reaches a point where he can no longer move forward in a task, and then demonstrate the next step in a way that the child will understand.

Keep Support in Place Until it is No Longer Needed

Remember, dealing with ADHD is not about the child understanding a specific task but is about them sustaining the mindset to do that task. This is an easy concept to understand in words but not so easy to remember in a given situation. For example, a child that is learning how to organize his room will understand the idea that books go on the shelves, toys go in the toy box, and clothing goes in the closet. Many parents may walk a child through this process several times, and once they see that the child fully grasps the concept and the importance of it, they remove their presence and expect the child to function independently from then on.

The problem with this is that the child has only grasped the fundamentals of what is expected but not yet learned it as a life habit. As soon as the parent pulls out of the picture, distractions can and will come in, and he will lose interest in the task. Ideally, parents will keep their support and presence with the child until they are sure that he has mastered the task and has made it a part of his regular routine.

Changes in Supervision Should be Done Gradually

Finally, when you do withdraw support, it should be done so gradually. As the child learns to perform each phase of a task independently, allow them that independence but remain close by in case, they need additional support. Many parents focus on an all or nothing approach which leaves the child floundering when a constant presence is no longer there. Once the child learns a specific task, step away for a moment or two and then gradually increase that time away until he is completely independent.

Of course, the preceding list of guidelines to use in preparing a working strategy for teaching your child is not a fool-proof system. Every parent will have to adjust their methods accordingly to fit the needs of their child. However, from understanding these basic concepts and how to work with an ADHD child, parents will be more relaxed having a basic understanding of how these affect the child and the benefits that can be gained.

Chapter 7: Giving Them a Workable Skillset

Every ADHD has a different set of challenges. Some may be lacking in emotional control while others may be struggling with organizational ability or flexibility. The best way to benefit your child is to address the skillsets he or she is weakest in. This can be done by taking advantage of those they are stronger in to help them to strengthen their own weaknesses.

Depending on the age of the child, your approach to this may vary. It is easy for parents to be overwhelmed by all of the things they must remember when dealing with an ADHD child but if they can keep in mind that teaching new behaviors starts with the external, then it may be easier to understand.

For example, a child that has repeated tantrums is very weak in emotional control. One of the first things parents want to do is modify the external environment. Think of all the external stimuli that could trigger an emotional outburst. This could be anything from the type of TV he watches to the number of people in a room. Watch your child and observe the triggers and then create a plan to remove them from his environment, and then gradually introduce them again in a step by step process so that he learns to accept them as he grows. This kind of adjustment in altering the environment rather than altering the child is much easier for the child to take and adapt.

The right change in the physical environment requires careful observation. If the child is having trouble with time management, you may need to keep him close by when performing certain tasks so that you can monitor and motivate when needed, you may choose to take them only to certain places where he is less likely to get off track when expected to complete an assignment or you might have to limit the amount of distractions to keep his mind focused.

If the child struggles with sustained attention problems, you will need to change his physical environment accordingly. The general idea is not only to teach the "task" she must do but also to teach the "executive skills" she is weak in. By doing this, you are building up your child's executive skillset to the point where she can eventually become independent of the need for constant supervision.

There may also be a need to adjust the social environment to build up skills as well. Children who struggle with emotional control, flexibility, or impulse control, it may require limiting the number of social interactions they encounter. They may only be allowed to play with friends for a certain number of hours, they may not be allowed to socialize until certain tasks are completed, or they may not be allowed to go to certain stores, shopping centers, or parks at certain times.

Which adjustments you make will depend largely on the triggers your child has but here are a few thoughts to get you thinking in the right direction.

Put up physical barriers for younger children and make certain areas off limits for older children.

Depending on the age of the child, physical barriers could include things like locking up certain items that are off limits; the alcohol cabinet, the car keys, the medicine cabinet are just some examples. It could also include placing fencing around an area the child is not allowed to enter or placing objects well out of the child's reach.

It could also include parental controls on the computers, television, or other technology; not allowing them use unless under direct supervision. Some parents may even password protect certain devices or applications to ensure their child has limited or restricted access.

Reduce Distractions

Distractions do not necessarily have to be in the same room with the child. Working in a noisy house, or outside noises coming in can have a negative impact on an ADHD child. While external noises and distractions may not always be under your control, creating a quiet environment may be key to helping them to master certain skillsets. In some cases, you may even be able to introduce positive noises and images to get the child to focus. Consider adding soothing music when it is homework time or white noise to drown out the more unpleasant distractions that may be out of your control.

Make Sure Their Life is Organized

It is much easier for a child to learn how to be organized if there is organization already in their life. They cannot learn to put things in their proper place if there is no place designated for it. Give them clear guidelines on how you expect things to be organized and what they have to do to achieve it. Some parents post a picture of how things should look and post it in their room, so they have a visual cue as a reminder of what is expected of them. Other children may benefit from a to-do list or a quality checklist to help them master this skill.

Give Them a Structure They Can Rely On

ADHD children need structure as they learn new skills. Rules and guidelines that are too loose can leave them floundering. Limit social interactions to a small number of people, have exact expectations outlined and make sure that games and activities have a beginning, middle, and end. The more structure they have, the more they will understand exactly what is expected of them and how they can succeed.

Change to Social Mix to Avoid Volatile Situations

As you become familiar with your child's social circle, you'll inevitably find some children that bring negative influences to your child. Don't be afraid to restrict their association with these children until they are more emotionally capable of handling them. This may mean cutting off some children (or adults) entirely, limit the amount of time they spend together or restricting association in certain environments.

Change the Nature of the Task for the Child

If it were left up to the children, everyone would do only the tasks that they find fun and exciting. However, this attitude does not reflect the world we live in. We often have to do things that we don't enjoy. This is called responsibility. However, for the ADHD child, it may be difficult to plow through these boring and mundane tasks the way they are presented to other children. The best way to ease them into doing these unwanted tasks is to make some adjustments so that they are more palatable.

There are a number of ways you can modify an unpalatable task. Here are a few suggestions but no doubt, you'll find other ways that may be more appropriate to your child's situation.

1. Shorten the task
2. Break the task up into smaller bite-sized pieces
3. Offer an incentive
4. Give them a checklist outlining each phase of the task
5. Make a schedule
6. Give them choices
7. Make it a challenge (perhaps play their favorite song and have them try to complete the task before the song is finished.
8. Make a game of it (beat the clock, finish before the timer goes off for example)

Adjust Your Interactions

As you come to better understand the importance of executive skills, you will naturally adjust the way you interact with your child. You will come to see just how important your role is in helping your child to master these skills. Adjusting your involvement before an exercise, during and after can help to impress on the child the importance of the skill you want them to learn. Consider these thoughts:

What You Can Do Before

Preparing the child for a difficult challenge can be very helpful. Some parents find it very effective to rehearse situations beforehand. If the classroom has certain rules about how supplies or tools are to be used, doing a little role-play on the way to school can be very effective in reinforcing the rules that they will have to remember.

Verbal reminders are also very effective in reinforcing lessons learned. Simple questions like 'remember what we talked about?' or 'what do you have to do next?' can help to keep the child on track.

You can also set up visual reminders when you're not there. Leaving little notes behind, sending them voice messages on their phone, or setting up alarm signals at times when things should be done can actually help the child to remember what is expected of him.

What You Can Do During

During an activity, you can give your child prompts to help redirect their mind to what they need to do. This might include a gentle reminder like 'what did we say you were going to do?' or a time-out to role-play the situation again.

If he has a checklist, you can also remind him to look at his list if he is struggling to remember what he is supposed to do. This is a way to transfer the responsibility from you to the child. By checking the list and grasping his next move you also give him the independence to execute an activity on his own.

Watch for triggers that can present an obstacle for your child. The more you understand the triggers that encourage unwanted behavior, the easier it will be to create a strategy to teach them how to overcome it.

What You Can Do After

Offer praise that fits the accomplishment. We have to always keep in mind that it is not just the task we want to praise them for but it is the mastery of the executive skills that will boost their self-esteem and motivate them to practice the skill more. So, rather than saying 'Good job on your homework,' be more specific in your praise. 'I'm really proud of the way you got started on your assignment without complaining.' or 'Thank you for not getting angry when your little brother was teasing you.' Make sure that the praise includes his attempt to master the executive skill you want him to develop.

Reviewing the situation can also be a tremendous help. Talk through the exercise step by step and together try to determine what worked and what didn't. Create a game plan that they can try to remember for the next time the situation arises.

Finally, you can get additional input from those who also interacted with your child. This could include other family members, teachers, and other school children. If a problem occurred getting an objective perspective from someone else can reveal how you can adjust your behavior or how to coach your child in the future should the situation arise again.

As we've already pointed out, working from the tangible to the intangible can be very effective when working with ADHD. Making adjustments to the external and tangible environment, whether it is physical or social will not automatically internalize the lessons they need to learn. However, if you are consistent in these lessons, eventually the child will be able to internalize them and make them a part of their normal routine.

But what happens when just modifying the environment is not enough? The answer to that question depends on several factors including, how urgent it is that the child master these skills, how much time you have, and the severity of the situation.

Addressing Behavior Issues

While modifying a child's environment works well when parents are with their children, it becomes more complicated when the child is outside the reach of your purview. Family members are usually the frontline of dealing with ADHD but asking a teacher or a daycare working to make exceptions for your child can be something else entirely. In such cases, the parents will have to prepare their child for the other environment by taking a more direct approach to teaching these executive skills. This can be done either through informal conversations with your child helping them to see the need for executive skills and giving them the tools to overcome obstacles that may come their way or it can be done with directly teaching them the skills they lack.

Teaching Them Informally

Informal settings are ways to teach your child without them even knowing. Parents use a teaching method called scaffolding to do this. It incorporates the method of providing just enough information to assist the child to succeed with one additional element; guidance on how to help them see how their behavior affects relationships or how to make the necessary connections associated with that task. It's a little like a scaffolding around a building; each level of the scaffold helps the child to reach another point in their advancement.

Verbal Scaffolding: Your approach to this will depend largely on the task, but you can verbally point out different aspects of the task making each new aspect a little more challenging than the first.

This type of teaching helps the child to build up their metacognition skills. Think of it this way. You're teaching your small child how to dress himself through a series of questions. You might first ask, 'what color is it?' Then you might point to an armhole and ask, 'what goes in here?' The child will answer my arm. Then you might ask the next question, 'what goes in here as you point to the other armhole. Once they understand the steps verbally you can walk them through the process finishing with a question like, 'what do you do now?' The child will answer button it. Continue this scaffolding until the child is able to complete the task on his own. After that continue to monitor his activity and interject only when it is clear that his attempt may fail.

Remember, use questions about what the child is supposed to do. Resist the urge to tell them what to do. This shifts the responsibility to the child and compels them to make decisions on their own. Avoid the temptation to make demands. Instead, try to explain why it's important. The hard rule of 'I'm the master of this household may work at times, but it does nothing to build up the child's level of confidence and self-esteem.

With verbal scaffolding you also want them to understand that you know how they feel. This can help to cement the bond between you and reduce the chances that the child will lash out in frustration.

Finally, it is important to encourage them to analyze their behavior after any given situation. Asking questions like 'can you think of something different you can try next time?' 'What are you going to do this fix your problem?' These types of questions help to build up their metacognitive skills.

Informal teaching can also be done with games or during family activities. In fact, parents seek to make every situation an opportunity to help their child to strengthen their weak executive skills.

Teaching Them Formally

There are times when a more formal and direct teaching approach can become necessary. This may be needed when the child has a profound deficit that requires immediate attention, and you may not have time to build them up gradually with the scaffolding approach.

Identify the root of the problem: This may not be very easy because the real problem is not always what you see. For example, a child complaining about doing his homework is not the problem you have to fix. The real problem may be he doesn't understand it, he can't concentrate, or his attention is pulled away by something else.

Establish a goal: Decide on the end result you expect to achieve.

Include the child: Always, when setting a goal, include the child in the process. The two of you should work on this goal together rather than dictating the result you expect. This helps the child to own up to the responsibility he has.

Decide on interim goals: No child will be able to go from zero to one hundred in one single step, especially one with ADHD. In setting interim goals, you need to start by determining what they are capable of doing now. Use that as a guide and build on it. If it takes thirty minutes to get them to sit down and start their homework then the first interim goal could be to do it in twenty-five minutes, then twenty and so on. By having an established baseline, you can make sure that each successive goal is only slightly more challenging than the one before. This requires that the child put forth extra effort but not so much that they are overwhelmed by the task.

Set a Time LImit: When setting a time limit, you need to have a baseline; you need to know how long it takes her to do whatever task she's given. Once you understand the amount of time it takes her, then you can set time limits that are within her range of ability.

Give Them a Voice: Sometimes they won't know how to express their level of frustration or anxiety. Give them a scale to measure how they're feeling. Some use a 5-point scale where one means they are doing okay and five is about as angry as they can get.

Make a Checklist: This gives the child something tangible to do as he works through the steps. It gives him a sense of accomplishment as he checks off each item on his list and it reinforces his efforts in working towards his ultimate goal.

Supervise: Once your child has grasped the fundamentals of her new skill it is important that you don't assume it is cemented in her brain. It takes time and repeated exercises before that skill becomes her own. This means that you have to continue to supervise her progress and be there to give constant reminders when she begins to forget from time to time. After a while, you'll find that you will need fewer and fewer reminders until she has mastered the skill completely.

While it may be challenging for both you and the child, in the beginning, your child will eventually learn and master these skills. One important fact to remember is that it takes time to reach the inner child within. The key to all of it is consistency. In order to ensure faster progress, it is necessary for you to not do this once or twice. It is an ongoing process, and it may take months, weeks, and in some cases years but it can happen with the right effort on everyone's part.

Chapter 8: Protecting Their Self-Esteem While Helping Them Grow

There is another extremely important part of training children with ADHD, and that is encouragement. After all, your goal is not to just get them to master a task but to get them to feel good about mastering it. One of the most damaging parts of anyone's psychological state is when words are used in the wrong way.

There is an ancient proverb that says, "A word spoken at the right time, oh how sweet it is." That expression fully encapsulates the power of the spoken word when it is used in the right way. Carefully chosen words cannot only motivate a child to work hard, but it can also inspire them to strive for higher levels. They will feel good about themselves and will do almost anything to hear you say it again. It is like gold to a child's ear.

Some parents, out of frustration will use force, ultimatums, and punishments to intimidate the child into better behavior. These types of actions are often based on the idea that the child is being deliberately rebellious and willful. As we've already learned, this is not the case with those who have ADHD. While punishment may be warranted from time to time, it is not the most effective way to teach. The focus is on the bad behavior and not the positive. It doesn't address the issue of teaching the child correct behavior but instead concentrates on teaching them what not to do. Add to that the fact that harsh words are painful and when they come from someone they are relying on getting them through life it is especially difficult to hear. In time, it drives a wedge between you, one that continues to grow separating you more and more each time they are shared. Eventually, you could find yourself separated from you child by a deep chasm that may be nearly impossible to overcome.

The best solution, therefore, is to you positive praise and encouragement to guide your child in the right direction. Praise given can do wonders for your child's self-esteem if done correctly. The easy way is to say words like, 'good job,' 'that's awesome,' or 'I'm so proud of you.' These are wonderful ways to start a positive dialogue with your child. However, studies have shown that when you are more specific, the praise yields the best results. Instead of 'good job,' try something like, 'I like the way you came in and started your homework right away, 'good job!' Now the child knows exactly what she is being praised for.

Even when you give praise, you have to be careful how you do it. Maybe you've seen those parents who mix praise and criticisms together. 'You did a really good job washing the dishes, why can't you do that all the time?' This kind of praise often confuses and frustrates the child rather than reinforces the spirit. At best, it reduces the power that your positive words are trying to say. Here are a few basic guidelines that can teach you how to give appropriate praise to your child when needed.

Teach Yourself to Pay Positive Attention

It may sound strange to tell a parent that they need to learn how to pay attention to their child, but that's exactly what's needed at times. Parents are often busy with affairs and forget to set aside one on one time with their children. Try to block out a time when it is just you and the child and observe them carefully. Don't hover over them like a mother hen but let them move about freely in their activity and watch what they are doing. If they are playing a game, don't jump in right at the beginning but sit back and watch for a while. Once you understand what they are doing narrate their actions back to the child, so they understand. This works better when you show a little enthusiasm in your descriptions. Match your enthusiasm to the age of the child. Younger children enjoy more animation, but you can tone it down as they get older.

As you speak, give them both verbal and nonverbal signs of approval when you see them doing something you like.

Non-verbal signs could include a hug, wrapping your arm around them, a pat on the head, a soft rub on the shoulder, a high-five, a smile, a wink, etc. Verbal skills could mean saying things like 'I like it when you do ….. Or 'that is so grown up when you do…..'

You can also praise progress. 'Last year you couldn't do ….. But now look at you.'

If during the course of your time together, turn your attention away and focus on something else. That usually works to get the child to adjust his conduct. If the bad behavior persists, tell them that your time together is over and that you'll spend time again when he can control his behavior.

Utilize the Power of Your Attention to Get Them to Comply

When your child is accustomed to your attention during relaxing periods you can begin to extend to other aspects of their lives. When you want them to obey a specific instruction first, give a clear command and then give immediate feedback narrating their behavior back to them. Once they have complied, leave them alone for a short period of time but return often to make sure they are still on track. Give praise where warranted and exit again.

Give only one command at a time so as not to confuse them and avoid asking questions or adding additional verbiage that could distract them even more.

Be Clear in Your Commands

When giving a command to your child, the compliance begins with you. Never give a command that you do not genuinely expect them to do. Back up every request with the reward or consequences outlined.

Do not make it in the form of a question as this can give them the idea that obedience is optional. Do not say, 'why don't you get ready for bed now?' rather make it direct, 'get ready for bed.' When you raise your inflection at the end of the sentence, children will subconsciously believe that you are asking them if they want to get ready for bed. Make sure your tone is clear enough to let them know you expect compliance.

You also want to make sure your child is listening to you. Eliminate all distractions that could divert their attention, and ask them to repeat the command, so you know they heard it and understood.

Teach Your Child Not to Interrupt

Children crave attention and will do anything to get it. If you give a lot of attention to a child that interrupts, you can expect to continue to have a parade of interruptions. To avoid this problem, before you are engaged in any type of activity like talking to a neighbor or on the phone give them a command to do something that will keep them occupied while you are otherwise engaged.

Make sure that the task you ask them to do is something they will enjoy. If the child obeys your instructions, stop what you're doing for a second to give him praise. Continue to do this every few minutes until you finish your activity. As the child becomes accustomed to this type of instruction and praise, you can extend the time between praises to keep them engaged.

If they look as if they're going to interrupt you, stop and give him praise for obeying what he's doing and then refocus their attention on the task you want them to do.

In the end, make sure you praise or reward the child for following your instructions before you go on to another activity.

Establish a Reward System

For children with behavioral problems, a reward system can be very effective in getting them to not interrupt you. Depending on their age and ability, you can give them an immediate reward for obedience, or you can set up a point system where they earn a number of points that they can accumulate for a larger reward later.

Use Constructive Punishment

When children become defiant or disobey, it is important to remember that it is not that they are refusing to follow your commands. Outright defiance is not a characteristic of ADHD. What is really happening is that their lack of executive skills often pulls them away mentally from whatever task you've assigned. It could be that the task is very boring, or very hard, which can be very uncomfortable for them.

Punishment, however, should be used as a last resort. It is better to find a more positive and self-edifying means of praise and incentives to motivate the child. There are several ways to punish a child in a way that helps them get the point.

Fines: If you used the reward system to motivate them you could also use the fine system to remove privileges. For example, if they receive 5 tokens for obeying your directives you can choose to deduct tokens for disobedience.

Make the Most of a Time-Out

Time outs can be very effective if done correctly. They must be place in an isolated place away from all distractions and interactions with other children. This can be very unpleasant for an ADHD child that craves distractions and stimulation. Make sure you give a clear command and set a time limit for them to comply. Make eye contact and use a firm tone of voice without yelling the instructions at them. Let them know in no uncertain terms why they are being taken to timeout and leave them there for the allotted time. Wait until the child is quiet and then repeat your command. If the child still does not wish to comply, then send them back to time out. If he complies or promises not to repeat the bad behavior, you can praise him for following your instructions.

If the child tries to escape, firmly put him back in the chair and repeat the instructions. If he persists, then you can give him a fine if you're using the point system or you can send him to another location void of all distractions. Make sure it is a place he cannot escape from.

Manage Your Child in Public Places

The secret to getting your child to be obedient in public lies in the preparation. Make sure he knows what's expected of him before you go out. Give him a short list of rules to follow and make sure he understands them. Have him repeat them back to you, so he owns the instructions. Review the instructions before you go in and if he disobeys take him out to your car and wait until he is ready to try again.

Establish an incentive to motivate him to obey your directives and a punishment if they disobey.

Keep them busy. Give them an activity that they enjoy to keep them occupied. As a matter of fact, it is a good idea to have several ready to go so you can keep them engaged while you are out.

No matter which methods you use to manage your child's behavior whether in public or at home they should be used consistently so as not to confuse the child. It will not be an easy ride, but if you are consistent, there is real hope that in the end your child will respond and grow from the experience. While it is easier said than done, never take a child's behavior personally or to the point that you forget you're working with a child with a disability. Learn the art of forgiveness for both your child and for yourself, and you'll both be happy for it.

Chapter 9: Bringing the Whole Plan Together

Now that we've covered some basic principles for dealing with a child with ADHD, you probably feel a bit more confident about the challenges ahead of you. However, it is a lot of information to take in and put into practice. You now must figure out how to put it all together.

There is no one-size-fits-all when it comes to parenting an ADHD child. Some parents work and are extremely busy while other parents may have more time but maybe struggle with ADHD themselves. In every case, there are positive and negative factors that must be weighed. Here are a few guidelines to help you to determine just how to make the best use of your time and energy while you prepare your child for the road ahead.

1. Do just enough to help your child succeed. Your goal is to make your life easier and still be able to help your child. Focus most of your efforts on those skills you child is weakest in and use their positive strengths to reinforce your lessons.
2. Learn the principals that the strategies are based on. In some cases, we gave you a blow by blow explanation of what each strategy is like, but as long as you understand and follow the

principal, you won't go too wrong. You've probably noticed that some strategies use steps that are repeated throughout the book. Your tone of voice, making sure the child understands the directive, consequences, and rewards, etc. That's because the same basic principles are used to create a variety of strategic methods. You can even use these principles to create strategies of your own.

3. Tackle the most frequent problems first and set the other ones aside for later.
4. Choose one skill to teach first. It may be tempting to throw the whole book at the child, but that will work against you. It is better to start with one or two tasks and build on that. It may take longer for them to master all the skills, but they will do so with more confidence and less frustration for everyone concerned.
5. Finally, include your child in the planning of their lessons. This will allow them to become a part of the process and motivate them to improve.

There is so much to learn and even more to be learned about ADHD, but at least from these recommendations, you have the platform from which to start. Keep in mind that your child may not completely overcome all of their weaknesses, but they will improve to the point where they can meet your ultimate goal, that of being functioning people in society.

Chapter 10: Giving Them Wings to Fly on Their Own

ADHD is not a condition that will eventually go away. Your child will have to struggle with this their entire life, so it is important that while you're training your child and teaching him the executive skills that they are lacking you remember that you are not just teaching a child but also a future adult to cope with life's problems.

Research has shown time and time again the often the successful adult comes from the successful child. You want your child to believe that they can succeed so do everything in your power to build up their self-esteem and praise then whenever it is warranted. This is directly connected to your relationship with them. The way you see view your child during their formative years is the way they will view themselves in their adult lives.

That's a powerful motivator for you to be careful about the way you interact with them. If they think you believe they are destined to failure, the odds are high that they will believe it too. This means you must walk a very fine line and keep your balance. Too much praise and help could strip them of their independence, compelling them to totally rely on others to help them and too little could discourage them to the point that they will stop trying.

Be extremely careful of how you label your child and the words you use when speaking to, about, or for him.

Never just decide for him but bring him in on the process. When they are able to take part in the decisions of their own life, no matter how small, they will be empowered and own up to the trust you have put in him.

Finally, foster creativity. As we progress further and further into the Information Age, many things in life are not as linear as they used to be. Your child may never be able to hold down a nine-to-five job, but they may find ways to support themselves nonetheless. Today, many artists, athletes, inventors, and entrepreneurs are successful because of their ADHD. It allows them to step out of the box and look at the world in a way that no one else can see it. So, just because your child's inclinations stray from the norm doesn't spell doom.

We live in a world that is changing at a rapid rate every single day. Always keep in mind that learning things can change at any minute. Every child's primary goal is to learn how to learn. The gadgets, devices, and technology used today may not be around when they are ready to enter the job market. Therefore teach your child the best way to learn for him. This way, he can continue to grow with the world around him and allow him to explore new ways to approach old problems. You might be surprised at what his unique way of thinking can bring to the world.

This is how you give your child the wings he needs to soar.

Conclusion

Thank for making it through to the end of *Identifying ADHD: A Guide to Cultivating Calm, Reducing Stress, and Helping Children Thrive!* Let's hope it was informative and able to provide you with all of the tools you need to achieve your goals whatever it may be.

While we have included lots of information inside we know we have merely scratched the surface of all there is to know about ADHD. Inside you've learned how to identify if ADHD is the problem with your child, what signs to look for, and how to know if you need to seek a diagnosis or not.

You've also learned how your relationship with your child can have a direct impact on his success. Positive interactions build up self-esteem in a child that is already struggling to fit in, and negative responses can be like a landmine poised to blow at any moment.

You've learned how to identify your child executive skills and determine which ones are weakest and then what to do about them.

We've given you some practical suggestions on ways to teach your child both informally and formally and the signs along with ways to measure their progress.

A step-by-step approach to teaching them to how to utilize the skills they have to accomplish just about any task.

No question, we included a lot of information in this book, and likely your head is probably spinning right now. Still, take your time and let your own mind absorb what's here and put it into practice. That way everyone will benefit from these guidelines and thus reap the reward in the process.

Finally, if you found this book useful in any way, a review on Amazon is always appreciated!

Description

When faced with the challenges of raising a child with ADHD parents can easily become overwhelmed. There are so many factors that need to be considered in identifying the disorder and knowing what to do. In Identifying ADHD, we strive to break much of this information down into bite-sized pieces so that parents can take a step-by-step approach to guiding their child to success.

Inside, parents will learn how to identify their child's strengths and how to help them hone on and fine tune those weaknesses. It then goes on to give them a practical, common sense approach to teaching a child with ADHD and gives them a simple foundation from which you can build up your child's self-esteem at the same time.

Parents are the primary counselors, teachers, motivators, and comforters for a child with ADHD so this simple yet easy to read tool at their disposal can prove to be invaluable for both parent and child.